Living Bipolar:
Learning to live with bipolar disorder

Sylvia Meier

Limits of Liability / Disclaimer of Warranty:

The authors of this information and the accompanying materials have used their best efforts in preparing this course. The authors make no representation or warranties with respect to the accuracy, applicability, fitness, or completeness of the contents of this course. They disclaim any warranties (expressed or implied), merchantability, or fitness for any particular purpose. The authors shall in no event be held liable for any loss or other damages, including but not limited to special, incidental, consequential, or other damages.

DEDICATION

This book is dedicated to all those in my life who live with bipolar disorder and me.

It's not easy being in my life, and I'm not always the easiest person to deal with but you all do so with such grace and compassion. I love you all and I hope even in my darkest of moments, and most difficult of days that you all know it too.

To my beautiful girlfriend, thank you for all your support, understanding and love. Without you I would never have reached where I am now. You are the shining star in my life, making each day move as smoothly as possible.

To my children, mommy loves you, even when she's a little crazy.

To all the other unnamed friends and family, thank you too. You all mean the world to me.

CONTENTS

Introduction:

Bipolar disorder is a disorder that can destroy the lives of those that it affects. As the afflicted individual you are not the only one who suffers from this disorder, in fact, all those around you suffer too. That doesn't mean all hope is lost. The fact that you are seeking information on bipolar disorder and trying to learn more about it shows that you have hope. You are seeking ways to ensure success with the disorder and to live with it, instead of losing your life to it.

Is there a cure? Short answer, no. Long answer, bipolar disorder is not something that needs to be "cured." It's a disorder that needs to be controlled. It needs to be managed and those who are living bipolar need to learn the proper techniques and skills to effectively manage, and live with bipolar disorder.

The hardest part about living with bipolar disorder is the mood swings. No one likes their lives manipulated and run by an illness and mismanaged, and untreated that is exactly what bipolar disorder can do. Instead, it is vital to learn how to control and minimize the ups and downs so that they rarely occur and when and if they do, knowing how to keep them under control.

Improving your quality of life isn't all the difficult. It does take time, it will take patience, and practice but that doesn't mean it cannot happen. With proper techniques and coping mechanisms you can live a healthy, happy, well regulated life. You have bipolar disorder, it doesn't have you.

Chapter 1:

Living Bipolar: It Begins With Understanding

A major goal for anyone who has bipolar disorder, is to live a normal life. That is, a life like those around us. One that is not controlled by mood swings, one in which you can get out of bed each day, and you know give or take how you are going to feel. A life where your day, and your entire life is not dictated by where you are in your cycle of mood.

The best way of course to learn how to live with bipolar disorder is to learn, and understand what it is, and what you need to do.

As with any treatment for an illness, there is no guarantee. Even if you go years with well maintained systems, you can fall off track and end up in the pit of depression or the upswing of mania. Speaking from experience, I can tell you that you can control your moods and your day to day life to a large extent, but there will always be extenuating circumstances that leave you slightly off-kilter. Learning more about your disorder, and yourself will help you have the greatest level of success.

To reach that point though, we must begin at the start, and that is an understanding of the disorder from a medical standpoint.

The Medical Side

Bipolar disorder is considered a mental illness, and like all mental illnesses it does have varying degrees. Just because one person with it cannot function and requires disability to live, doesn't mean that you or any other person who has bipolar disorder cannot be successful and happy in life.

Like all mental illnesses though, it does require medical intervention. As much as you may wish and pray it didn't your medical team can become your greatest assets. Having others to help support you, and understand your disorder can help you reach your best level of success. We will get back to that though.

In the past bipolar disorder was referred to as manic depression and in many ways that name is more fitting, as it describes the two major ends of the spectrum that someone with the most severe of the disorder can experience. Mania and depression. What we've learned is that manic and mania style behavior is only one extreme end of this condition. The other part of it is that of depression. And both have varying levels, such as hypomania, and mild depression. Learning to cope with these extremes and everything in between is vital to your well-being or the well-being of your loved one.

Thus far, the cause of bipolar disorder is unknown. It is believed that there is both a genetic factor to it, as well as environmental but there is still no confirmed cause.

For most people bipolar starts when they are just in their

teens. Some believe that it is triggered by puberty or the trauma and hormones associated with it. Others will not develop this condition until they are in their early adult years. And of course, as with any disorder or illness, there are those outside the norm, who present the symptoms at a very early age. No matter when it is diagnosed or presents itself, one thing is certain, bipolar disorder lasts your life time.

Now, this is where bipolar disorder can get kind of tricky. You see with most disorders and illnesses, you present with symptoms all the time. With bipolar disorder, you can go into what they call remission (which is a term I thoroughly despise) in which you are showing no symptoms at all. You are level, well managed and not swinging between mania and depression. Your moods also remain in the realm considered "normal". Of course, for the vast majority, and especially those untreated or without a treatment plan that covers all aspects, being level and without the extreme swings is highly unlikely.

In all reality, if you do not get treatment for bipolar disorder, it can take you out on both ends of the spectrum. With mania your inhibitions tend to go out the window and you end up in risky, ill advised situations which can cost you your life, and with depression, suicide becomes a very enticing way to end it all.

The biggest thing you need to know about bipolar disorder, and something I fought for years myself, is that you NEED medical intervention. You NEED to seek help, and do your very best to adhere to the advice, stick to your medication regime and learn all you can about yourself and how bipolar disorder affects and alters your life.

Am I Bipolar?

This is commonly the first question in your quest. Am I bipolar? And I challenge you from the get go to rephrase that in your mind. You see, you are NEVER your illness or disorder, and the disorder is never you. Instead, in a more positive and enhancing light you should be asking, do I have bipolar disorder? The starting point for this is to learn about and understand the symptoms. A word of caution here. If things are so bad that you are in danger of harming yourself or those around you, stop reading and please seek immediate medical attention. Situations like that cannot and will not be solved by reading a book. They require the attention of those properly trained to deal with your immediate needs.

To start, one needs to understand that the majority of symptoms play in some way or another to the emotional stability of a person. Bipolar disorder though a mental health illness, can also be considered an emotional disorder. They way moods present themselves in the afflicted individual is very telling.

They alternate from states of mania. Mania is a point in which a person is euphoric. Not just happy but through the roof with euphoria. They also tend to have a sense of invincibility. Nothing can knock them down, they cannot be killed and no risk is too high. (More on these later)

The low side of emotions are episodes of depression. Like mania isn't just being happy, this depression is not just sadness. This is the type of sadness that keeps you in bed, makes you idolize death, and feel as though the entire world and future is futile and nothing will ever be worth living for or good again.

Due to the fact that bipolar disorder is somewhat of a spectrum disorder (people can have all sorts of levels of capabilities and symptom severity) the intensity of these highs and lows can and will vary from person to person and from one episode to the next. For some, the symptoms can be quite mild but for others they can be quite severe. In addition to this, you may also have very normal times too. These times are typically referred to as periods of remission.

When you are manic, you may feel or exhibit to others (often only others will see your behaviours, which is why support, which is talked about later is so important.) and or even all of the following:

- You may feel extremely happy and optimistic. Not the normal, I can handle this optimism. More along the lines of nothing can go wrong or ever will go wrong.

- You may feel euphoria. This is a crazy high. It's not happiness, it's not elation, it's beyond that.

- You may also have an inflated self esteem or ego, too. You can take on the world, the world bows down to you. You get the point.

- You may have very poor judgment, and you may know this by being told by others that you've made the wrong decision. Alternately, when the episode is done, you may find that you made a great many choices you would not have otherwise made, or done things very out of character for you.

- Your speech can be very fast. It's almost like someone has turned up the speed on your speech to the 2 times or faster. (I've seen and heard myself when I was manic and hypo-manic and just the sound of how quickly I am talking wears me out.)

- Your mind is going crazy with thoughts. Know those times when you just cannot get your brain to turn off, it's the middle of the night, you want nothing more than to sleep but all you can keep thinking about is, well, everything.

- You may become agitated and even snappy. This is one of those symptoms others may be better indicators of then yourself.

- Physical activity may be increased, too. Ever spent 2 in the morning cleaning your house, well cooking all needed meals for the next day? The manic me has many a times.

- Many will be aggressive in their behavior, often more so than is needed for the situation. This is one of those times where you become a danger to yourself and others. Your aggression can get you into fights and even trouble with the law and or authority.

- Sleep deprivation is a big one. And it's not an issue that would bother you. In fact, you may feel that sleep is simply wasting time you could be spending doing the millions of things your racing mind is thinking of.

- You may have problems with concentrating on what you should be doing. You may be easily distracted, and have problems getting tasks accomplished. Or you are hyper-focused and able to complete massive tasks, in a time frame unreasonable for the task at hand.

- You can be reckless or you may take chances on things that you normally would not do. This one can be a very bad one. You may become promiscuous to the point of endangering yourself. You may spend money without thought of what it is actually needed for. You may find yourself walking a very dangerous path, with impaired judgment.

As mentioned before, there are essentially two states to bipolar disorder, one being mania, which we just discussed, and the second being depression.
The depressive bipolar symptoms include:

- Feeling very sad, very guilty or feeling that all is lost. Not just a small sadness either, or a justified one. Just an overall deep seated sadness with little to no origin.

- Hopelessness is a common feeling during a depressive episode. The feeling as though nothing can or will ever get better and even that there is no hope for tomorrow or reason to live for today.

- You may be very tired even to the point of not caring about getting anything accomplished. In fact, while mania makes you feel like you don't need any sleep, depression makes you feel like all you need to do is sleep.

- You may lose interest in the things that you do on a regular basis. Those things that you did everyday. Even the things that you once loved and enjoyed doing.

- You may be very irritable, losing your temper for no real reason.

- Another symptom can be pain without cause. If you've ever seen the commercials about where depression hurts, and the answer being everywhere, it is very true.

- The most severe and possible deadly of all symptoms is suicidal idealization. That is a fixation on ending your own life. This is one symptom that you need immediate help for.

If after reading all of this it sounds like you, first don't be afraid. There are many people who have bipolar disorder that go on living life with it, and being quite successful at it all. There are many famous people who did their very best work during manic states. Secondly, realize that getting a diagnosis and help is vital. You need to talk to a doctor and begin the process to feeling better, and living life with stability.

What Causes It All?

Anyone with an illness or a disorder may find themselves asking why me? How did this happen to me? What caused this all? I should've, could've, would've.

Of course, as of right now no one can answer that. The cause is unknown. There is no known cause only some ideas of what could cause it to manifest in a person.

Many believe that it is a combination of factors that lead to this condition including environmental, genetics, and biological factors. Doctors believe that these conditions not only cause the onset of bipolar in people but also control when the episodes that you experience happen and how frequently they do. It includes things like the stress and trauma experienced in your life, the environment you are raised in, or live in and the list goes on.

All that is known so far is that those of us that have bipolar have problems within the brain.

There are chemical messengers in your brain that go between the nerve cells and the brain itself relaying information. These are called neurotransmitters.

In those that have bipolar disorder, those messengers are somehow different and simply communicate in a different way to the brain triggering the symptoms that we face.

It is believed that those of us that suffer from bipolar have something in our genetic codes that makes us react and exhibit the symptoms that we do. While this genetic disposition doesn't per say actually trigger the condition to happen, those that have this coding actually have a better chance of developing it at some point in their lives. This is where the genetic link comes in and why, it is very likely that if you have bipolar disorder, someone else in your family does and that your children could be at risk for it as well. When I say at risk for it, it doesn't mean they will get it, simply that they have the probability of getting it due to their genetic coding.

In addition to this genetic code, most doctors believe that it is necessary for you to have some environmental effects to happen in order to trigger the problem. This can include such things as drug abuse and very stressful events. Sometimes, a very traumatic event especially those that are psychological can trigger bipolar.

If you ask someone who has been formally diagnosed with it about prior life traumas you will find that a vast majority of them have it. That's not to say that everyone who presents with the symptoms and the disorder underwent a traumatic experience in their lives, simply that it is highly likely.

What Are The Risk Factors To Bipolar Disorder?

Family history is huge. If you have someone in your immediate family that has been diagnosed with bipolar disorder or any form of depression you are in a higher risk category of having bipolar disorder, or the genetic coding for it then someone whose family has no history at all.

Again, if you have genes that are passed down from those in your family that have these abnormalities, then you are more likely to experience bipolar. While the exact genes are not know just yet, there are many researchers working on finding the gene that makes you more or less likely to have bipolar disorder.

Calling In The Pro's?

If you're still reading along you probably realize by now the importance of getting medical attention and treatments for your, or your loved ones, bipolar disorder. The problem is though, that many who have bipolar disorder do not realize they have it, or see a problem with it being untreated. I know it wasn't until I was properly medicated and in treatment that I realized just how different things were from the pre-treatment me and the newly found post treatments emotionally stable me.

Of course you may realize that something is just not right, but not realize the severity of the disorder in it's entirety. In addition, you may not realize just how difficult the mood swings can be not only on your body and mind, but on those who love and support you.

Therefore, it often takes someone else, or a severe episode that brings you to the attention of the law or medical community before attention is ever sought for a diagnosis or help. This is also why if you are a loved one reading this, that you help your loved one get help for the disorder.

If you do not seek help, or help your loved one seek help, things will simply continue to get worse, till you or your loved one can be severely hurt, emotionally or physically, or worse, end up dead.

Which Doc Is The Right Doc?

Now that you are ready to take the step of seeking medical help, the question becomes which doctor is the right doctor. The first doctor you should speak to is your family doctor. They are the ones to get the ball rolling and get you moving in the direction of living healthier, and more stable.

Oftentimes, the family doctor will then refer you to a psychiatrist. Don't be afraid. I was terrified the first time I saw one, now I am grateful that I did.

Try not to worry; the process of seeking help in dealing with any type of mental illness including depression and bipolar syndrome is quite simple to do. Take a loved one with you that has noticed the symptoms that you are experiencing.

The first thing that your doctor will ask is what type of symptoms you are having. He or she will ask you to describe both the depressive symptoms and the mania symptoms.

During your first meeting with the doctor, you'll talk about your daily life, the episodes you are experiencing and your overall health. The first thing that he or she will do is work on ruling out other medical problems and other mental health problems. Other conditions, such as mood disorders, attention deficit hyperactivity disorder, schizophrenia, and even a personality disorder, can have similar symptoms to bipolar conditions.

Your doctor may also ask you to undergo tests that will determine if there are any other things that may be causing your condition. They will need to find out if you have physical causes contributing to your bipolar disorder.

Now this is where most people can get nervous and wonder what the rest of this stuff has to do with a diagnosis of bipolar disorder. One of the things that will be discussed and asked about is substance abuse. Your doctor will ask and need an honest opinion about this. If you drink alcohol, use illegal drugs such as marijuana and cocaine, then you need to tell your doctor about these things. Remember, your doctor can't talk about this with anyone else. These types of drugs can alter the mood and in some people create larger fluctuations of moods. They can also lead to an overall destabilization of an individual with bipolar disorder, and they can confuse and interrupt and even at times escalate the symptoms you are experiencing.

Another possible reason for your mood swings can be due to health problems like thyroid disorders. Here, a blood test will be required. It will test how well your thyroid is working. Many that have mood swings actually have an under active thyroid. The good news is that if this is the problem, there are medications that can treat thyroid problems and you may not have bipolar disorder at all. Another reason for the blood tests is because some of the medication used to treat the disorder can affect kidneys, liver, and other organs so checking their pre-medication state is vital.

Still there is more to talk about with your doctor. You'll want to tell him about the medications that you are taking, as these can also cause a number of mood swings. For example, medications like corticosteroids can cause mood swings. If you are being treated for depression with medications, or for anxiety, then your medication can lead to mood swings. The medications that are used to treat Parkinson's disease are also mood swing prone medications.

Your doctor will ask you about your diet, too. The foods you eat lead to the number of nutrients that you get. Those that are lacking in B 12 vitamins in particular can experience vast mood swings.

Any of these types of conditions can lead your doctor to determine that you are suffering from bipolar disorder. By talking with you and looking at the test results that are given to you, your doctor can determine exactly what is happening with you.

It is very important for you to communicate with your doctor about any of your needs and to be honest about your condition. By telling them about your daily life, including the bad parts, he or she can make the right decisions to help treat your conditions. Anything you withhold or are not entirely truthful about can interrupt any progress you may make, or alter the type of treatment you are given.

Once all the initial questions and conversations are completed and the blood work and tests are finished, you are started on your road to treatment, and stability.

During the time that you wait to see a psychiatrist or other specialist, your family doctor may ask some tasks of you. This could be a simple as keeping a mood diary (which tracks sleep, eating, and obviously moods over a period of time) to even starting on some preliminary medications to help stabilize you till you begin seeing what will become your primary medical team.

Sylvia Meier

Chapter 2:

Why Should I Get Help Anyway?

Bipolar disorder is a mental illness. It is not like a cold or flu that given time will just go away. It is not like a broken leg which will heal on its own. Without the attention of a professional, bipolar disorder can and will get worse.

What happens to you will be unique. My story is unique to me as well. There is no way of knowing if your condition will worsen quickly or at all. That said, the majority of us who have the disorder at some time or another reach so far gone that we require hospitalization. Even I have spent my time in a psychiatric ward.

If you have bipolar, just like most mental illnesses, other conditions and the environment you live in can make it even worse. For example, if you are trying to deal with anxiety, you will have a hard time doing so because of the bipolar disorder. In conditions where this is life threatening, for example if you are suffering from alcoholism, this can be a very serious problem.

If you can't keep yourself from consuming alcohol then your life may be in danger. I myself avoid alcohol at all costs. It is simply not worth it to my stability and mental well-being. Not only will the alcohol cause problems for your health, but your bipolar disorder can make you think irrationally and even cause you to put yourself in dangerous situations. A good example is me getting on a plane, despite a major fear of heights and flying across the continent to meet someone I met online! For this reason, seeking help is a must.

For some, the length of time between depressive symptoms and mania symptoms can be very short. You can move from one symptom to the next quickly, leading to confusion and even health scares. This rapid cycling in itself will cause you quite a bit of grief. In fact, rapid cycling can be one of the most dangerous states you can find yourself in. You move so quickly between states that even if you are trying to stabilize yourself on your own, it will get out of hand rather fast.

It can get even worse, too. It is possible, believe it or not, to be in a state of depression as well as in mania at the same time. When this happens, the end result is that your mind and emotions are completely wrapped in each other. You are agitated and annoyed. You are unable to sleep or eat. You can't get your thoughts to be organized. This is a mixed state. Ask anyone who has ever experienced it and they are sure to tell you it was beyond horrible. And to those around them, it is costly and frightening.

Even worse, when this happens, people are more likely to think about suicide. This can be very dangerous because people in this state of mind are not thinking rationally at all and can make the wrong decision. The majority of suicides occur in this state. When you are manic, you don't tend to idolize suicide or death. Your behaviours may say otherwise and may ultimately cause your own death but that would not be the intent. When you are depressed, you are often too tired or listless to carry out plans of suicide. When you are in a mixed state though, all odds are off. You have the energy, the motivation, the plan, and the capabilities of following through with them. If you ever find yourself in a mixed state or feel you are entering a mixed state, it is of utmost importance you talk to your medical team or even go into the emergency room. It is that dangerous.

Another problem is that of psychosis. Bipolar symptoms that combine both mania and depression symptoms can lead to psychosis. This is a very serious mental illness in which your personality is completely disorganized. You are impaired with what is real and what is not. You are hallucinating and you are delusional. Even those that very strongly believe in things can end up making decisions the other way. You can and may lose all sense of morality, and your own personal character. Psychosis is not something to be toyed with or taken lightly. It is possibly the most severe of all bipolar states.

Living Bipolar: The Danger Of It

Even beyond the physical risks that you place yourself under when you face and live bipolar are the just as devastating effects that it has on your relationships. It can take such an extreme toll on relationships that oftentimes, the person who has bipolar disorder finds themselves very much alone and isolated.

Many people with bipolar will have trouble holding onto relationships. They may move from one person to the next quickly because of the mood swings that they deal with. In addition, those that are suffering from bipolar often times make mistakes with dealing with others. They simply are confused as to what the true emotion is supposed to be during any such situations. Another complication to relationships and bipolar disorder are thing like hyper-sexuality; impulse control, or lack there of, and a simple instability of emotions and dependability.

In addition to this many with bipolar also have financial problems to boot. They do not make the right decisions regarding money, spending on credit and making choices in products. With this comes a number of problems from having to file bankruptcy to having to burden other family members. A manic person can spend money without any thought or reason, thinking that tomorrow doesn't matter, only today does. This can lead to draining your life savings, making stupid decisions like quitting your job, selling your home or just running away and living recklessly.

Even a depressive episode can do the same just a different way. Instead of the disregard for tomorrow, it could be done to try and cheer yourself up, make yourself feel better, or because you have plans on when you'll take your own life, so the money, the house, the savings will be of no use to you at that point.

Still, one of the worst effects of bipolar is the way that people who have it treat themselves. Many find that the only way to cope with what is happening to them is to isolate themselves from everyone.

Self esteem, and self hatred can play majors roles in your life. Having to cope with and deal with situations that have arisen because of behaviours or things you did when you were in an altered state of mind can be quite difficult and take it's toll on your self image. With that, the changes in your body, and physical appearance that can occur swinging between episodes can make a large impact on your self esteem as well.

How others view you also comes into play with your self image. You may have friends who you tend to associate with only when manic and so when they see the depressed side of you they don't understand, think you changed (which you in fact have) and no longer are interested in spending time with you. Losing friends, or having fair weather friends is something I have come to understand and realize is par for the course with this disorder. I figure though, now that I am healthier, if someone cannot handle me during my worst times, they don't deserve me during my best.

During depressive phases especially the isolation can become severe. This is doubly bad when you are having a severe episode. Without the protection and support needed from a loved one, you can all too easily let suicidal thoughts take control. Because of this isolation, it is important for those that have loved ones in this condition to provide them with the care that they need to keep them safe.

As you can see, the complications of bipolar disorder can be quite severe. Because many people that suffer from this condition simply do not realize that they have it, it can easily escalate and even put people in danger just doing the things that they do everyday.

Just simple everyday tasks like driving can become dangerous and an issue if your mood alters. Driving fast and reckless is easily done, and regularly done when manic. Drifting attention and simply not caring can be very dangerous when depressed or focusing on ending your life by any means.

Going out and partying can become an excessive dangerous thing. Many people can get by with having a drink or two at a party and knowing to call it quits. Manic me could drink the room under the table and not care. I would consume inconceivable amounts and concoctions of alcohol, without any concern on how my behaviours were becoming or my total and utter lack of awareness and judgment.

These scenarios can be played out with many other day to day situations in your life too.

Getting help though, thankfully, can really improve your outlook on life and reduce your risks and complications significantly.

Chapter 3:

Living Bipolar: The Doctors Treatment Plan

As we've discussed, the first thing that you need to do is to talk with your doctor to determine what is affecting you and get your diagnosis. If it is in fact bipolar disorder, then there are several treatment options that your doctors will recommend to you. Or you can pursue on your own.

The process of treating your bipolar disorder will come from two main forms, from your doctor that is. The first is that of medication. This is a given starting point for anyone with a diagnosis of bipolar disorder. This does not mean you will be medicated for the rest of your life, simply that you will be medicated and stabilized while other treatments and plans are looked at for the long term. Of course, for others, depending on the severity of their disorder, it could be something that is needed on a long term even lifetime basis.

The second form of treatment is that of psychotherapy. The combination of these things has been effective in helping millions of people to improve their lives even while living bipolar.

There is no cure for bipolar, but with the right treatments for the condition, you can increase your quality of life and keep yourself safe, too. And personally, I wouldn't want a "cure" living bipolar is very much a part of what makes me, well me. I wouldn't want to be any other way (now that I'm stable that is.)

It is the combination of these two treatments that will ensure you have the most success in the long run. Medication is great for stabilization when you're in rough shape but it doesn't help you learn to cope, or give you the tools you really need to be successful at overcoming and living bipolar.

Medications

I won't really go to in depth here as medication is something that should really be discussed with your doctor, and the knowledge that everyone reacts differently to medication. What works for one person may not work for the next. What is great for one person, may destabilize or make another person quite ill.

The main purpose of medication is to help keep you stable. When you're up and manic it helps bring you down, when you're heading down it helps hold you up. It is the stability most of us simply don't have on our own.

There are many different types and uses and there are actually some medications now that actually have bipolar disorder treatment as an on label use. For the most part though the medication that you will be prescribed is for off-label use but don't let that worry you, all of mine are off-label medications and they work wonderfully for me.

Psychotherapy

Psychotherapy, the word itself can sound terrifying, but in reality it is anything but. It can be one of the most important factors in dealing with and eventually living with bipolar disorder.

During psychotherapy, you and your doctor will work together to determine the best possible treatment for you. Usually, you'll be taking medications during this process. Medications don't work all by themselves, it does require more treatment types in order to ensure your success. Medication can of course be the start of your treatment plan but should never be the only part to your treatment plan.

By meeting with a doctor to talk about psychotherapy, you both can learn more about your bipolar condition. The goal will be to find patterns in your episodes. This can also be done with mood charting. Which is why your family doctor may have asked you to start one when you were first being referred to a psychiatrist. It helps move your treatment further forward, quicker then waiting for your first meeting with the psychiatrist. So what's the point of mood charting? By tracking and exploring the pattern of episodes that you go through, your doctor and you can better understand what triggers them.

By tracking your mood changes, the doctor can see if there is something that causes them in the first place. These are called your triggers. For example, if you take medications for some other condition, those medications may actually be triggering your mood changes and leading to the effect of bipolar. Other things can include changes in sleep pattern, stress and even the weather outside! Yes, the seasons themselves can affect your bipolar disorder.

Of course the knowledge of the triggers is great, but that is not enough. You and your doctor need to work out ways that once you know your triggers you can cope with and deal with them. For myself, I know that summer and more sunlight tends to bring on the manic side of me and winter brings out my depression. To help cope, in the winter I use light therapy to ensure I am still getting enough of what I need to stay out of a deep depression, and in the summer I am more cautious and open with friends and family looking for signs of mania or hypomania.

By learning your patterns, triggers and eventually coping mechanisms for them you will be better prepared and able to live a stable bipolar life.

Medication is great in helping stability, but psychotherapy is the real life saver in it all. Understanding your disorder, what causes you to do things and how your moods work is essential to your success. It will also help keep you grounded when you think you are so stable as to stop taking your medications.

When you truly have understanding of your disorder and your behaviours and how grave it can be not to take your medication or follow your treatments you'll learn that taking that little pill each day and staying within your limits in other parts of life is key, for you'll understand the damage you create in your life and the lives of those you love otherwise.

What's Right For You?

Learning what's right for you can be a frustrating process. Finding the right cocktail of medications, the right therapy and treatment plan can take time and a lot of patience. I went through years, yes years, of trial and error to find my precise medications and treatments that worked for me. In the end it will be very much worth it all.

You need to also remember to be very open with your doctor

about any and all issues. If you are having medication issues or side effects, talk to your doctor. They are there to work with you and help get you on the right track.

Chapter 4:

Living Bipolar: Why The Struggles?

Giving up should never be an option for anyone living with any illness or alive for that matter. Although medication and psychotherapy are methods for dealing with bipolar disorder, many times individuals simply will not take their medications or follow their therapy plan. They stop. They give up. They simply can not stand the entire process of fighting their bodies and minds. They just give up. I've done this myself. Was fighting the illness, was trying to stabilize and stopped it all. Said enough of the medications, I don't need them. It didn't end well.

As you can probably imagine, this is simply not the best route for you to take when it comes to caring for your condition. Yet, a vast number of bipolar us will experience this feeling at some time or another. Why is that? Those that take anti-psychotic medications and mood stabilizers are often the types of medications with the most side effects and therefore the most commonly stopped by the patient.

Yet, those that just stop taking these medications against their doctor's recommendations often face a huge problem. They relapse. What was a stable condition, once again worsens. What was under control, spirals out of control once again. Hospitalizations begin. You may experience homelessness, victimization, and even be involved in various types of crime. You may wake up to find yourself either in jail or in a hospital. Chances are without medications and treatments you need you'll end up in trouble.

Why then would anyone stop taking their medication?

Well, even those who do not live bipolar and take medication everyday will face this from time to time. You take your medications for so long and suddenly things are good. You feel like you no longer need to take them, after all, all your symptoms are gone, things are under control. Forgetting to take into consideration that the reason things are that way is the medication itself.

A key thing to understand here though is it doesn't mean stopping all your medication is going to cause problems. Even stopping just one can do it. When you are non-compliant in your treatments, you can and may end up suffering because of it. Just because you feel good doesn't mean you don't still have bipolar disorder, and the only reason you may be feeling as well as you do is the entire cocktail that you take. Remove one medication and you have essentially changed your cocktail and things may no longer be as good, or as stable.

In the end though, this does not cover all the why's simply, what can happen.

There are many reasons behind the why's of struggling with living bipolar.

I Don't Understand My Illness!

Not fully understanding the illness can be a big one. Without fully understanding what makes you do or act how you do, you'll never really be able to understand the full impact not taking your medication or following your medical advice can have on yourself and those around you.

You see most of us simply take the medication because the doctor says to. We don't question him or her on why we should take it, or what it does for us, simply that since we were told to take it we should.

Therefore one of the most important things we can do for ourselves and our loved ones is to be informed and stay informed about bipolar disorder, as well as the medications and treatments we receive for it.

Dependance On Other Things

Dependency on other drugs or even alcohol can also cause severe issues and non-compliance. If you cannot drink because of your medications but want to go out and party and have a good time, you may stop taking your medication so that you can drink. This complicates the issue because now you are no longer medicated and are consuming a mind altering substance. An extreme recipe for disaster if ever there was one.

For me I had to make the choice. Was an occasional drink worth missing my medication? Was drinking and partying worth the issues that arose from missing medication? Was the behaviours that became very apparent from my drinking worth it. Or was the better option not to drink at all. And luckily I had the insight into myself and my illness to know the latter was the better choice.

Instead of deciding not to drink or do drugs, the addiction that many bipolar patients have to these substances keeps them consuming those instead of medications. This can be very detrimental to their well being, though. For this reason, it is essential that patients pair medicinal treatment with substance abuse treatment at the same time in order to stop themselves from these types of situations which can ultimately lead to an even worse health crisis.

Ugh, I Can't Stand My Doctor!

Hating your doctor or not seeing eye to eye with them can be another reason for non-compliance. I had this issue myself with a psychiatrist. I didn't like her, we clashed from the get go and so for me it was a case of why should I listen to you when you won't even listen to me. Eventually, I realized that I shouldn't neglect my health because I don't mesh with my medical team. So I fired her and got one that worked with me instead of against me.

You don't have to see everything 100% the same as your doctor but you need to be able to have at least a working relationship with them in order to fully understand and help yourself and get the most from your time with them.

The end result of that interaction is important. No longer was I putting my own health at risk simply because of a personality clash with a health care professional. You need to feel comfortable with those taking care of you. If you don't you need to stand up for yourself and for your health and get someone who can do the job.

Outta The Way, I Gotta PUKE!

Side effects are a major contributor to non-compliance in medication. Who wants to force a pill down their throat only to vomit moments later, or all day from that pill. Or gain 60 pounds, or be unable to sleep, or lose their sex drive. And the list goes on. Side effects can be scary, they can make you sick as can be, they can make you feel like you've lost your damn mind. Why then, when there are so many side effects would anyone want to continue using medication?

Sometimes, and more often than not, the usage of the medication and what it changes in you, is more important than a side effect. See, here's a perfect example. New medication took it first day, found myself on the side of a major road throwing up. Try again, same result. Next day, forget it, not happening and I became non-compliant in my medication. Here's the important lesson here though, I called my doctor up and said, hey this is what's happening, this won't work for me, can we look at something else. And so we are. I could have been like many others who have probably had this side effect and went, I'm not taking it. Never mention it to the doctor and wondering why things aren't working how they should be.

It is so important to be honest and open with your medical team. They are there to help you and only you. The only person you are cheating by not being open with them is yourself and your loved ones. You need to be open if you're not taking a medication so you can find something that works for you.

Or in the end it could simply be the dose is wrong. You never know. There is no straight, laid out rule about what will work with bipolar disorder. It is very much trial and error, and we unfortunately are the guinea pigs in our own search for stability.

Denial, Denial, Denial. It Can't Be Bipolar Disorder!

Why would you listen to a doctor and take the recommended medications if you didn't believe in your diagnosis. Of course you'll be non-compliant. You're not going to ingest a medication for a syndrome or illness you don't have. That simply would not make any sense.

Denial is something we all go through. No one wants to be told they have a mental illness. No one wants to realize that they will probably take medications for the rest of their lives. No one wants to really have that label attached to them.

And of course, there is a major stigma attached to mental illness. Why would you want to become a part of that group. Why would you want to identify yourself as one of them. You know those crazy people...

I Love Myself

Another reason for non-compliance of medication and treatments is simply because you love the manic phases. Getting well meant no longer having those crazy times in my life. I felt for the longest time if I was medicated and stable I would no longer be me. Truth of the matter was, manic and depressed I was unable to be me. I was letting my bipolar disorder rule my life and me. I wasn't living bipolar disorder, it was living me. It controlled me. Looking at it this way made it that much easier to accept that yes, what I did and who I was manic is a piece of me, and what I did and who I was depressed is as well, but in reality, the real me, is the stable me that floats somewhere in between those two states.

Chapter 5:

Living Bipolar: Learning To Live

One of the biggest things you need to take away from this book is that you can change your life. You can learn to live with bipolar disorder instead of allowing it to live your life for you, or destroy it. You can learn to cope and deal, and live on a day to day basis. It's not always easy, it's not always hard, but in the end the effort you put into it is more than worth it. After all, you only have one life to live, make it worth it.

Of course you could also be of the other mind frame that you don't need to worry about it. What happens will happen, but I think we've covered pretty well what can and will happen if you don't take hold of your bipolar disorder and instead allow it to take hold of you.

Now, that you realize that, take the time to realize what changes you can make in your life to actually improve your overall quality of life.

Don't try to make all of these changes today. Give yourself time and patience to work through each one. Doing so will give you more ability to actually be successful with coping with bipolar disorder.

In this chapter, we talk about a number of simple ways that you can improve your quality of life by learning coping techniques. Take them one step at a time but try to get them all worked into your lifestyle. They seem simple because they can be just that.

Sleeping Like A Baby, Or Not!

Believe it or not, the way that you sleep plays a significant role in your bipolar condition. What's important to remember here is that when you sleep in a normal pattern, there are chemical changes in the brain that are beneficial.

Simply get enough sleep each night, but do this by going to bed about the same time each night and get up about the same time each morning. Creating a sleeping pattern like this will improve your symptoms.

If you work a job that has you sleeping strange times of the day, you need to try to work out a schedule so that even when you are not working, you are still sleeping the same times of the day. This is essential to your coping skills. It also gives your mind the time that it needs to clear and to wake up refreshed.

In fact, when you do need to make changes in your sleep pattern that are drastic, such as a new time zone, talk to your doctor about the best way to do this without causing problems for yourself.

Monitor Your Medications

We've talked a lot about taking the medications that you need to take and the reasons for doing so. But, you can also learn to cope with this process to make it that much more successful for you.

Take your medications even if you feel great. Do what your doctor tells you to do in regards to taking them even when you have no symptoms. Even if you feel really good, that's your medication talking and working! By stopping the consumption of them, you simply allow the symptoms to begin all over again.

To make the entire process of medication taking easy plan out your schedule so as to include your dosing. For example, when you wake up in the morning, have your breakfast and take your morning pills. If you take a second pill later in the day, do so after dinner, for example. By pairing medication taking with meals, for example, you keep yourself from forgetting them.

If you do take more than one pill and are easily confused by them (and who wouldn't be?) purchase a pill organizer and use this to portion out your medications. Those that are for a week or even a month at a time are excellent tools to insure that you don't forget and don't become confused with medications.

Another tip to remember about your medications is that they don't mix well. If you get a cold, consult your doctor about which cold medications you can take with your bipolar medications. I've learned the hard way the cold medications make me go hypo-manic to manic very quickly. I know this in advance, as do my loved ones so they help me stay grounded when and if I need to take cold medications. You should never mix them with any type of alcohol or other drugs. If you are using either, talk to your doctor. They can help. They are there to help. Don't keep it to yourself and wait for disaster to strike.

If another doctor prescribed medications for you, don't take them until you are fully sure that they are aware of the bipolar medications that you are taking. If and when medications are mixed, they can interact with each other and even bring on extreme conditions including health crisis like events.

Healthy Bodies, Healthy Minds

Part of managing bipolar disorder is to completely organize and regulate your life in the best way that you can. For those that are used to working very hard, every day, this may mean pulling back some to a normal paced activity level.

No matter what you do, by regulating the amount that you do the same or about the same each day, you also help to ease those chemicals in your brain and therefore avoid the symptoms that can sometimes happen when you are frantically running around one day and doing nothing but watching television the next day!

This can also help you identify when you are going manic or depressive. If you do the same amount of activities and things each day and have a fairly regular routine then find yourself worn out from doing it or unable to keep up with it, it could be an indicator that you are going into a depressive cycle. Likewise, if you do the same amount of activity each day and one day find you've done all your days activities before noon you may need to watch that you aren't hypo-manic or even manic.

Knowledge really is everything with this illness and the more you know about yourself and the illness the better your ability to cope with life and all that comes with life will be.

Support, Support, Support!

Getting support from your family is vitally important. Many of us like to think that we can do it on our own. That manic side of us hangs on through it all and tells us we are invincible, we don't need others help to deal with our illness. But, as we've discussed, it is very difficult to do this. Most of the time, you won't realize how severe your mood swing is. You may not realize that you are lashing out at a loved one for no reason. A lot of the time, you need those in your support group to be the ones to tell you that hey, something is not right, or that your mood is swinging the other way again.

Step one then is understandable. It is to tell those that you love about your bipolar disorder. As difficult as that sounds, those close to you can be your safety net. They can help you to realize what is happening and how you are acting. A supportive person will guide you to help and will stand by you through this prognosis and this life long challenge. I was afraid in my most recent relationship to tell her that I had bipolar disorder, but I also realized in order to have a relationship with any sort of intimacy and closeness I needed to be honest. So I opened up and told her and it was the best thing I could have ever done. She is and has been my biggest fan and supporter from day one.

Step two is to realize that you aren't the only one that is suffering. We often lash out at those that we love. Those in your family have to deal with mood swings that can be quite severe. Although you feel you can't do much about this, helping your loved ones to be educated and informed about your condition will reduce the amount of stress that plays along with bipolar disorder.

If they know what you are suffering from, they can help you. If they don't, they don't understand why you are doing what you are doing. That leads to family stress and painful situations. Without an understanding of what is happening, your family just can't be as supportive as they could be otherwise. And that can lead to a breakdown of your family, and even more stress, causing an even worse situation to arise.

In addition to just having knowledge of the effect that bipolar disorder has on you, you should also seek out the help that you need from a family therapist. Even a family that doesn't have much strife in it will need to get the help and support of a therapist. Bipolar disorder causes trauma in families and having this additional help is a saving grace in the way of understanding. Helping those you love come to terms with and understand your illness will go great lengths to helping you and your illness and stability as well. By properly equipping those we love with the tools they need to be around us, we can better love ourselves and be that healthy, happy stable person we are striving for.

Finally, when an educated family can support the person that is suffering from bipolar disorder, he or she can strive for improvement with help. The family can provide support when mood swings take over.

And, they can help to keep you and your doctor informed about the way that you react to situations, to mood swings and even to your medications. That adds up to a successful situation for the bipolar disorder patient.

The family unit is a tool that all bipolar disorder patients need, but many times you may feel the desire to simply run and hide. You may feel as if you would rather be alone. Getting through that feeling will lead to success.

In the end, the more open you are about your illness the better equipped those who love you will be. And the better equipped they are, the better the situation is for all involved.

STRESSSSSSS!

Just reading the title of this section you are thinking to yourself that you can't do it. You've heard it before. You know that stress is a killer of many people, not just those that suffer from bipolar disorder. Yet, it is essential that you look at your life and identify those times when stress has lead to mood swings or even out of control behaviors that put you at risk.

Consider this. If you push yourself at work to be the person that does the most, what do you accomplish? You probably will cause the onset of numerous symptoms of bipolar disorder specifically that of mood swings. When this happens, you put yourself in a position of not being able to work or even worse putting your position at jeopardy.

Therefore, you end up not actually benefiting from all of your hard work, but instead have fewer benefits and ultimately you drop the productivity level that you could have had.

On the other hand, if you would have worked a steady schedule and done what you should have done in regards to stress management, you ultimately would have accomplished more.

Here are some tips for stress management at work.

- Work the same hours as much as possible. By working a predicable and steady schedule allows you to stick to a schedule which helps to lessen mood swings.

- Get the rest that you need. You need to try to sleep at the same time each day. You need to be able to monitor your sleep patterns to reduce mood swings.

- When you are suffering from mood swings, consider whether or not you should be working. For some, it may mean talking with your doctor about how they affect your job. Ultimately, you need to decide if you are benefiting yourself or not by continuing to work and tough out these mood swings.

- Take time off. Those that take time off often improve their overall health and well being. By getting time off each week and even vacation time, (or taking time off when you need to) you improve your level of stress and how the body reacts to it.

- Don't work in overly stressful environments. While you may not feel that this is something that you can control, it needs to be. Those that suffer with bipolar need to consider their health above anything else. Mood swings, depressive and manic symptoms, can be made worse when you put yourself in a position to deal with a lot of stress.

- Work through problems. If there are small things that happen that cause you to worry or cause stress, handle them right away. Small problems turn into large ones that are much less likely to be dealt with. By handling problems quickly, you reduce the stress toll that they take on you ultimately.

Reducing stress should be one of the most important things that you do. By doing so, you lessen the risk of having a mood swing because of stress. Learn to spot stressful situations and learn how to get out of them effectively! It will pay off.

Also knowing your own limits is important when dealing with stress. One situation that won't stress someone out, may be the most taxing stressful situation to the next person. Know yourself and don't compare yourself to others. Simply trust what is right for you and use that to judge the situation, not what others say, or what they suggest should or shouldn't be a stressful situation for you.

Watch For It, It's Coming...

Believe it or not, learning to watch for signs of the onset of mood swings can be an excellent tool to aid you in coping with your illness. The early warning signs of an episode can be seen before they become full blown swings.

Why do you want to actually pay attention to this? There are a number of benefits that can come from you seeing and taking action when you see them.

Unfortunately, your doctor can only give you an idea of what will happen to you during a mood swing. That's because each person is unique and that in itself provides for challenges. Each person will move from depressive symptoms to manic symptoms differently and at different times.

The faster you notice that your mood is changing, the faster you can take action to prevent it or at least to deal with what is coming. The faster you do this, the faster help can get to you. This is also why it is so important to have support and honesty with your support group. They may notice well ahead of when you do and be able to clue you in sooner rather than later.

What are the warning signs? Here are some things that can be a small mood change that ultimately can be a predictor of a large mood swing behind the next door. Learn to notice these to spot mood changes.

- **Sleep changes.** If you are on a sleep pattern (which you should be) when you notice that you can't sleep or you are tired even after getting a full nights rest, this can be a predictor of a mood swing.

- **Energy level.** Fluctuations in energy levels are a strong indicator that you are having a mood change. Since most of the time mania will incorporate increased energy while depressive symptoms take away, you can see how this could be spotted.

- **Loss of sexual interest.** Some patients will encounter times when they don't want any type of sexual touching. Although it is common for people to be interested and not interested normally, a change that is significant should be noted. With mania you can also see an increased sexual interest.

- **Concentration.** You go to work and get the job done. Sometimes, you may have a feeling that you just can't stay on task. When you feel that you can't concentrate and finish the tasks that you started, this can be a sign of a mood change.

- **Self esteem.** It is important for family members to take notice of these situations. If you or your loved one determines that you are down and out or you are saying negative things about yourself, then this could be a sign that depressive symptoms are coming. It is essential that these things be spotted and treated as soon as possible. The manic me has wicked self esteem. She can and will take on the world. The depressed me is the quite the opposite. If I feel either of these coming on it is a pretty good indicator that I am shifting my mood.

- **Thought changes.** If you just for no reason seem to be very optimistic, or you are thinking about death a lot, this can be a sign that you are having a mood swing. If these thoughts turn suicidal, it is imperative to seek help as soon as possible.

- **Changes in the way you appear.** Some bipolar disorder patients will go through stages in which they feel as if they need to change the way that they look. You may change the way that you groom or to the level that you groom. You may all of a sudden hate the clothes that you have. These can be signs of a mood swing because of the emotion that is often attached to them. Manic me hates the way I look. Hair cuts, clothing style changes the whole works indicates Miss Manic and her moods are making an appearance.

The early warning signs of a mood swing can be wonderful tools to aid you in spotting trouble before it happens, or at least to the degree that it can happen. But, one of the problems with this is that most people can't spot these things on their own. They often see these stresses as just their everyday lifestyle.

For this reason, it is important that family members be able to spot these early warning signs and then help you to get through them. By spotting changes in you, your family can help you to get some help and quickly!

What should be done if you experience some of these mood changes? If you notice the warning signs, you should contact your doctor as soon as possible to find the relief that you need. He or she can offer supportive help that extends to medication if he deems it necessary.

This also can be helpful in spotting patterns of mood swings and that can be a tool to long term treatment as well. This is also where the mood diary can come into play. If you chart your moods over extended periods of time, months and years you will see more and more patterns emerge and be better able to understand and know when to expect the changes and how to better cope with them and live bipolar.

Here's What's Up Doc

Although you may hate to go to the doctor and you may think that your doctor never has anything good to say, it is very important to keep him informed. By telling him what is going on and what you are feeling, he can make better decisions for you.

You should contact your doctor:

- When you feel that a mood swing is going to happen sometime soon.

- When you feel that you are experiencing a mood swing

- When your medications are not working the way that you thought they were supposed to

- When you have any type of suicidal thoughts, feelings of despair or are having trouble getting through the day without feeling sad.

- When your family members tell you that you are going through a mood swing or they tell you that you are showing signs of either mania or depressive symptoms due to their understanding.

Your doctor can help you to learn to cope with these situations. They can also prescribe medication differences that can also act as a tool to improving your health and well being.

By keeping your doctor informed, you allow your symptoms to be monitored. Your doctor can learn patterns and even notice the things that trigger these episodes to happen. That can lead to benefits throughout your lifetime including the avoidance of those situations which will lead to fewer episodes throughout your lifetime.

Learning to cope with bipolar disorder is a must. By taking a look at your life right now, you'll be able to see things that can be changed that will ultimately improve your well being. Do you sleep right? Do you eat right? Do you know what your early warning signs are? Taking care of these changes now will ultimately improve your overall well being.

You can learn to cope with bipolar disorder. You can learn to live with it too.

Chapter 6:

Living Bipolar: Support Is Success

Prior to my suicide attempt I had joined my first support group. I was scared, I was nervous, I had no idea what to expect or why I was really doing it, all I knew is that if I was to move forward I needed support to do it, and what would be better support than others out there living bipolar.

Perhaps, right here, right now as you read this you are actually considering that you could use more support in your life but you don't know where to start, how to look for it or even what you should expect from it. Let's start by understanding that walking in with no expectations is the best way. You never really know what you'll get from a group until you start going to it and learn the group dynamics and what you really want out of the support group.

Support groups aren't magic, but having enough support in your life that truly support you can change and alter your life. It can make it worth it. It can make it better. It can help you to learn to better cope and live with bipolar disorder.

Learning to live bipolar is not easy. Learning to live without illness is not easy. It can be challenging and it will be challenging. That does not mean that you cannot do it though. You can and will be able to do it. One of the keys to success though is having the support to get through what life throws your way.

Support groups can be just what you need. They are none judgmental. Many if not all of them will be living bipolar as well. It's not your doctor, your spouse, your children. Just another human being living bipolar who is able to relate to what you are living through and what you are doing to try and overcome it all. Being with others going through the same issues as you can make you feel less alone. They can give you perspective that others without bipolar disorder may not be able to. It can be the very best support you never knew you needed.

Who Is Your Support Group?

Support can come in many forms and you may be surprised at how much support you really have or the lack of support in your life.

Support can come from your medical team of course, and they should be a key aspect in your support team. They support you with your medications, they support you with therapy and all other methods of treatments in your overall health plan. They are not the only support you have or need through.

Friends and family can play a vital role, but the key to this is that they know what is going on with you. If they don't know that you are living bipolar, or that you are having issues coping or need support, they may be lacking in their ability to assist you with support. They may only have partial knowledge of the situations and be unable to help altogether.

Letting them into your world can be tough, but letting my girlfriend know right off the bat about bipolar disorder was one of the best thing I could have ever done. She has held my hand at the psychiatric ward and wiped away my tears, she has attended support groups with me, she has asked me when I'm a little off if I notice the mood change, or if I am doing alright, and this has been a life-saver. She often catches the mood shifts before I do now, and that is the type of support we all need in our lives.

Or, of course, they can be the opposite spectrum and not believe in mental illness or your diagnosis. My family fell into this category. One of the best things I did for my life and illness was realizing that they were toxic support. People telling you to just pull yourself together or just get over it aren't helping your situation, in fact, they could be making it that much worse. You need support who is just that, supportive. Not ones that cut you down, call you out and make coping even more difficult.

While having friends, family and your medical team is great, sometimes we need more. Sometimes we need people who are completely outside the situation to be able to talk to, confide in and find support in.

This is where support groups really come in.

Groups that meet to discuss living bipolar either in a professional capacity, or simply as a meeting place where all involved have bipolar disorder can be an essential key in your support group. As I spoke of before there is something different that you get from a group of people who all are learning to live and cope with their own disorders and able to help share their own issues and insights.

Isolation is one of the worst things you can do with bipolar disorder. Pulling away from the world can kill you, literally. Not having people around you to check up on you, for you to talk to, for you to confide in and get help from can lead to disaster. You need to be comfortable in life, and hiding away scared of your disorder is no way to live and can lead to suicide.

Ask your doctor, check Google. Do whatever you have to to get the support you need. You need to take care of yourself and support is essential. You can live with bipolar disorder but it takes a team to make it. This isn't a solo fight.

There are others out there fighting the same battle and sharing war stories will be the most comforting thing you do. Once you realize you are not alone, you are very much apart of a larger group, you may understand that many live normal functioning lives and you can make your symptoms tolerable and do what it is you want to do with your life.

Conclusion:

It may be hard to swallow and harder to cope with but your illness, bipolar disorder is not going away. It is something that you and I will live with for the rest of our lives. Some days will be tough, no matter how good you've gotten at living bipolar. Other days you will forget you even have it and somewhere in the middle there will be days where you know you have it, but you are too busy living life to care. Hopefully, in the end, once all skills are in place this is where you find yourself.

The more you learn, the more you cope, the more you get out there and start living life, the sooner you will be living bipolar instead of dying or suffering from it. It's not the easiest path, but in reality, there is no path in life worth living that is.

You can do this, you can succeed at it. And hopefully now, with some more information, some coping skills, and life skills, as well as building your support group you will be able to have the standard of living your deserve to have instead of one dictated by an illness.

Coming to terms with my illness was one of the best moments of my life. From that point on I was able to begin living. I hope sharing my story, and this little book helps you do the same. Check out the about the author for more information.

ABOUT THE AUTHOR

I'm not doing this about the author is traditional fashion. It's awkward and plain strange to write about myself in the third person.

My name is Sylvia.

I'll be 32 this summer.

I am the mother of 5 beautiful children.

I am the partner of the beautiful woman who has been my greatest support in my fight.

I am living bipolar. I have bipolar disorder type one. I was first diagnosed at 13 years old, and went through the typical denial and rebellion.

Fast forward 17 years and life is off-kilter, all sorts of wrong, my illness has left my life shattered, tattered and my life on a string.

Suicide attempt, stopped by myself was the best and worst moment of my life. It was the wake up call I needed, and the scare I needed. I took my illness in my hands, decided to be in control instead of my disorder being in control and here I am a year later in the best mental health of my life.

I won't lie, there are days that are tough, there are days I long to be manic again. Overall though, I am happy, I am healthy and I have more support in my life than I could ever imagine.

I am a writer by passion. This is not my first book and surely will not be my last. I am in the process of writing another one called "Woman Broken, A Child Lost" which is about my life, my struggles and everything in between. It too will hopefully be out this year, but is one of those stories that will not be released until perfection is reached as it is my story. My full story.

Till then you can always find me and support for yourself on my website which is my story and writings as well. Check it out at http://www.MyBipolarWorld.com

In the end, I send you all much love and hope. If you take nothing else from all of this at least know you are not alone, and if you ever need that ear, feel free to contact me at my site. I do my best to respond to everyone as time and living bipolar allows.

Love,
  Sylvia

www.ingramcontent.com/pod-product-compliance
Lightning Source LLC
Chambersburg PA
CBHW070614290526
45790CB00002B/907